# Reduce Your Inflammation

## The 10 Proven Secrets to a Transformative Anti-Inflammatory Diet

Beginner Recipes, Meal Plans, Lifestyle Tips to Cut Pain, Boost Energy, Revitalize Health

Dr. Jeff Gerbers

# Table of contents

**Introduction** ........................................................................... 4
    The importance of an anti-inflammatory diet ........................ 4
    Overview of the "10 Proven Secrets" .................................... 6
    How this book can help you achieve a healthier lifestyle ........ 8

## Chapter 1 ............................................................................ 11

**Understanding Inflammation** ............................................. 11
    Definition and causes of inflammation ............................... 11
    How diet influences inflammation ..................................... 14
    Long-term effects of chronic inflammation ......................... 19

## Chapter 2 ............................................................................ 23

**The 10 Proven Secrets to a Transformative Anti-Inflammatory DIet** ................................................................. 23
    Secret 1: Incorporate Anti-Inflammatory Superfoods .......... 23
    Secret 2: Focus on Omega-3 Fatty Acids ............................ 24
    Secret 3: Hydrate and Choose Anti-Inflammatory Drinks ..... 24
    Secret 4: Eliminate or Reduce Inflammatory Foods ............. 25
    Secret 5: Optimize Gut Health for Better Immunity ............ 26
    Secret 6: Spice Up Your Diet with Anti-Inflammatory Spices ... 26
    Secret 7: Embrace Healthy Fats ......................................... 27
    Secret 8: Adapt Portion Control and Mindful Eating ........... 27
    Secret 9: Incorporate Regular Detoxification ...................... 28
    Secret 10: Combine Diet with Lifestyle Changes ................. 29

## Chapter 3 ............................................................................ 30

**Beginner-Friendly Recipes** .................................................. 30
    Breakfasts ........................................................................ 30
    Lunches ............................................................................ 44
    Dinners ............................................................................ 61
    Snacks .............................................................................. 78
    Desserts ........................................................................... 91

## Chapter 4 ............................................................................ 108

**7-Day Meal Plan** ................................................................ 108

## Chapter 5 ............................................................................ 111

**Lifestyle Changes to Complement Your Diet** ..................... 111

Exercise routines suitable for all levels _____111
Stress management techniques _____112
Importance of sleep and how to improve sleep quality _____113

## Conclusion _____115

# Introduction

## The importance of an anti-inflammatory diet

"In today's fast-paced world, where processed foods and stress have become the norm, the prevalence of chronic inflammation has significantly risen, becoming a silent threat that contributes to numerous health issues ranging from mild discomfort to serious diseases. It's here, amidst this backdrop, that the anti-inflammatory diet emerges not just as a dietary choice but as a transformative lifestyle, pivotal for restoring and maintaining optimal health.

Chronic inflammation is the body's prolonged response to harmful stimuli, such as toxins, infections, or poor dietary choices. Unlike acute inflammation, which is a beneficial part of the body's healing process, chronic inflammation can lead to a myriad of health problems, including heart disease, diabetes, arthritis, and various autoimmune conditions. It can also have a profound impact on energy levels, mood, and overall vitality. This is where the importance of an anti-inflammatory diet comes into sharp focus.

An anti-inflammatory diet is more than a set of dietary restrictions; it's a proactive, holistic approach to nourishing the body with foods known for their healing properties. This diet emphasizes the consumption of whole, nutrient-dense foods—rich in antioxidants, omega-3 fatty acids, vitamins, and minerals—that work synergistically to reduce inflammation, bolster the immune system, and enhance overall well-being. By incorporating an array of colorful fruits and vegetables, lean proteins, healthy fats, and whole grains, this diet stands as a powerful tool against inflammation.

The transition to an anti-inflammatory diet is not merely about avoiding certain foods that trigger inflammation but about embracing a food philosophy that celebrates variety, balance, and the intrinsic joy of eating for health. It's a journey that invites us to rediscover the natural flavors and textures of real food, to listen to our bodies, and to make mindful choices that support our health and happiness.

Furthermore, this diet is not a one-size-fits-all solution but a flexible, adaptable framework that can be tailored to individual needs, preferences, and health goals. It's about making informed, conscious decisions that prioritize long-term health over temporary convenience or indulgence.

By choosing to follow an anti-inflammatory diet, you embark on a path of self-care that transcends the mere act of eating. It's a commitment to a lifestyle that nurtures the body, mind, and spirit, offering a holistic approach to reducing inflammation and enhancing quality of life. This cookbook, "Reduce Your Inflammation: The 10 Proven Secrets to a

Transformative Anti-Inflammatory Diet," is designed to be your guide on this journey. It will unveil the secrets to a diet that can not only reduce inflammation but also revitalize your health, boost your energy levels, and bring about a profound transformation in your well-being.

As we explore the tenets of this diet, beginner-friendly recipes, and lifestyle changes, remember that each step taken is a step towards a healthier, more vibrant you. The power to reduce inflammation and revitalize your health lies in your hands, and with each meal, you have the opportunity to nourish your body in the most profound way. Welcome to your transformative journey towards an anti-inflammatory lifestyle."

# Overview of the "10 Proven Secrets"

The "10 Proven Secrets" form the core of our anti-inflammatory diet approach, designed to mitigate inflammation and enhance overall health. These secrets encompass:

1. **Anti-Inflammatory Superfoods:** Prioritizing nutrient-dense foods that naturally combat inflammation.

2. **Omega-3 Fatty Acids:** Emphasizing the importance of omega-3s in reducing inflammatory responses.

3. **Hydration and Anti-Inflammatory Drinks:** Maintaining optimal hydration and incorporating beverages that support inflammation reduction.

4. **Reducing Inflammatory Foods:** Cutting down on foods known to trigger inflammation, such as processed and sugary items.

5. **Gut Health:** Focusing on gut-friendly foods to support a healthy immune system and reduce inflammation.

6. **Anti-Inflammatory Spices:** Utilizing spices with powerful anti-inflammatory properties in daily cooking.

7. **Healthy Fats:** Selecting fats that contribute to heart health and help manage inflammation.

8. **Portion Control and Mindful Eating:** Encouraging mindful eating practices to prevent overeating and its inflammatory effects.

9. **Regular Detoxification:** Incorporating detoxifying foods to assist in eliminating toxins that can cause inflammation.

10. **Diet and Lifestyle Changes:** Advocating for a combination of dietary adjustments and lifestyle modifications to maximize the anti-inflammatory benefits.

This summary outlines the strategic dietary and lifestyle shifts advocated in this cookbook to combat inflammation and promote a healthier, more vibrant life.

# How this book can help you achieve a healthier lifestyle

"This cookbook is not just a collection of recipes but a comprehensive guide designed to steer you towards a healthier lifestyle. By focusing on the principles of an anti-inflammatory diet, this book serves as a beacon for anyone looking to mitigate inflammation, enhance their energy levels, and revitalize their overall health. Here's how it can help you achieve a healthier lifestyle:

**Personalized Approach to Nutrition:** Understanding that every individual's body responds differently to various foods, this book offers a flexible approach to an anti-inflammatory diet. It provides the tools and knowledge needed to tailor your eating habits to fit your personal health goals and preferences, encouraging a more mindful relationship with food.

**Educational Foundation:** Before diving into the recipes, the book lays a solid educational foundation about inflammation and its impacts on health. This knowledge empowers you to make informed decisions about your diet and lifestyle, understanding the 'why' behind each recommendation.

**Diverse and Delicious Recipes:** With an emphasis on diversity and flavor, the recipes in this book are crafted to make healthy eating enjoyable and sustainable. From hearty breakfasts to nourishing dinners, each recipe is designed to be accessible to beginners while also appealing to seasoned cooks looking for new inspirations. These dishes showcase how an anti-inflammatory diet can be both satisfying and delicious.

**Practical Meal Plans:** To ease the transition to an anti-inflammatory lifestyle, the book includes practical meal plans that simplify the process of planning and preparing healthy meals. These plans are designed to reduce the overwhelm of changing dietary habits, making it easier to maintain these changes long-term.

**Lifestyle Integration:** Recognizing that diet is just one piece of the wellness puzzle, the book also explores lifestyle changes that complement the anti-inflammatory diet. It covers the importance of regular physical activity, stress management techniques, and the role of quality sleep in reducing inflammation. This holistic approach ensures that readers are equipped to improve their health in all aspects of their lives.

**Community and Support:** Finally, this book aims to create a sense of community and support among its readers. It encourages sharing experiences, challenges, and successes in adopting an anti-inflammatory lifestyle, fostering a supportive environment for making lasting health changes.

By integrating the "10 Proven Secrets" into your daily life, "Reduce Your Inflammation" offers more than just a dietary change; it presents a transformative journey towards a more vibrant, energetic, and healthy lifestyle. Whether you're dealing with chronic inflammation or simply seeking to improve your overall health, this book provides the guidance, tools, and inspiration needed to make lasting changes."

*Chapter 1*

# Understanding Inflammation

## Definition and causes of inflammation

"Inflammation is a fundamental biological process that the body uses as a protective response to injury or damage. It is the body's way of signaling the immune system to heal and repair damaged tissue, as well as defend itself against foreign invaders, such as viruses and bacteria. While inflammation is a vital part of the body's healing process, when it becomes chronic, it can lead to a multitude of health problems.

### What is Inflammation?

In simple terms, inflammation is the body's attempt to protect itself with the goal to remove harmful stimuli, including damaged cells, irritants, or pathogens, and begin the healing process. The classic signs of acute inflammation include redness, heat, swelling, pain, and loss of function. These signs are evidence that the body's immune system is responding to a problem and trying to fix it.

However, inflammation can be classified into two main types: acute and chronic. Acute inflammation is a short-term response with localized effects, typically beneficial, leading to healing and recovery. For example, cutting your finger might become inflamed briefly but heals within a few days. Chronic inflammation, on the other hand, is a long-term, often less intense response that can persist for months or even years. It can result from the failure to eliminate the cause of an acute inflammation, exposure to a low level of a particular irritant over a long period, or an autoimmune response to normal tissues.

## Causes of Inflammation

The causes of inflammation are varied and can be a response to several factors, including:

- **Pathogens (germs) like bacteria, viruses, or fungi** When the body detects these foreign invaders, the immune response is triggered, leading to inflammation as the body attempts to neutralize the threat.
- **Physical injuries or trauma** Cuts, scrapes, or any form of physical injury to the body tissues can induce an inflammatory response as part of the healing process.
- **Chemicals or radiation** Exposure to certain chemicals or radiation can cause tissue

damage, leading to inflammation as the body tries to repair itself.

- **Chronic stress** Prolonged stress can lead to an imbalance in the body's ability to regulate the inflammatory response, often resulting in chronic inflammation.

- **Poor diet** A diet high in processed foods, trans fats, and sugar can provoke an inflammatory response in the body. Conversely, a lack of anti-inflammatory foods like fruits, vegetables, and omega-3 fatty acids can also contribute to increased inflammation.

- **Lack of exercise** Regular physical activity is known to reduce inflammation, whereas a sedentary lifestyle can increase inflammation levels in the body.

- **Obesity** Fat cells, particularly those in the abdominal area, can produce pro-inflammatory molecules, contributing to chronic inflammation.

- **Autoimmune diseases** Conditions like rheumatoid arthritis, lupus, and inflammatory bowel disease (IBD) are characterized by the immune system mistakenly attacking the body's own tissues, leading to inflammation.

- **Environmental factors** Pollution, exposure to allergens, and secondhand smoke are environmental factors that can trigger inflammatory responses.

## The Impact of Chronic Inflammation

Chronic inflammation is at the root of many diseases, including heart disease, diabetes, cancer, arthritis, and bowel diseases like Crohn's disease and ulcerative colitis. It's also linked to conditions such as obesity, asthma, and even mental health issues like depression and anxiety. The persistent, low-grade inflammation characteristic of these conditions can lead to significant tissue damage over time, as the body's immune response attacks healthy cells and tissues instead of just harmful invaders.

Understanding the causes and mechanisms of inflammation is crucial for developing strategies to reduce its impact on the body. This knowledge forms the foundation for the rest of this cookbook, guiding you through dietary and lifestyle changes that can help manage and reduce inflammation. By recognizing the signs of inflammation and understanding its causes, individuals can take proactive steps towards mitigating its effects and improving their overall health and well-being."

## How diet influences inflammation

"Diet plays a pivotal role in either exacerbating or alleviating inflammation within the body. The foods we consume can significantly impact our inflammatory processes, affecting overall health, energy levels, and susceptibility to chronic diseases. This section explores the intricate relationship between diet and inflammation, highlighting how certain dietary patterns can provoke an inflammatory response, while others can offer protection and promote healing.

Pro-Inflammatory Foods

Certain foods are known to trigger or worsen inflammation. Regular consumption of these foods can lead to or exacerbate chronic inflammatory conditions. Key pro-inflammatory foods include:

- **Refined Sugars and Carbohydrates:** High intake of sugar and refined carbs can lead to a spike in blood sugar levels, prompting an inflammatory response. Foods high in added sugars, such as soft drinks, candies, and baked goods, as well as white bread, pasta, and other refined grains, are common culprits.
- **Trans Fats:** Found in some fried foods, fast food, commercially baked goods, and processed snacks, trans fats can increase levels of harmful LDL cholesterol and trigger inflammation.
- **Saturated Fats:** While not all saturated fats are harmful, excessive intake, particularly from

processed meats and full-fat dairy products, can contribute to inflammation.

- **Omega-6 Fatty Acids:** While omega-6 fats are essential in moderation, an imbalance in the ratio of omega-6 to omega-3 fatty acids can lead to inflammation. Many processed and fried foods contain high levels of omega-6 fats.

- **Processed and Red Meats:** Certain chemicals in processed and red meats can lead to inflammation, especially when consumed in large amounts.

- **Alcohol:** Excessive alcohol consumption can cause inflammation and damage to the liver, digestive system, and beyond.

Anti-Inflammatory Foods

In contrast, a diet rich in anti-inflammatory foods can help reduce inflammation, improve immune function, and lower the risk of chronic disease. These foods contain various antioxidants, polyphenols, and nutrients known for their inflammation-fighting properties. Key anti-inflammatory foods include:

- **Fruits and Vegetables:** Rich in antioxidants, vitamins, minerals, and fiber, fruits and vegetables (especially those brightly colored) can significantly reduce inflammation. Berries, leafy greens, and other vegetables like broccoli and Brussels sprouts are particularly beneficial.

- **Omega-3 Fatty Acids:** Foods high in omega-3 fatty acids, such as fatty fish (salmon, mackerel, and sardines), flaxseeds, chia seeds, and walnuts, can reduce the production of inflammatory substances.
- **Whole Grains:** Whole grains contain fiber, which can help lower levels of C-reactive protein (CRP), a marker of inflammation in the blood. Examples include quinoa, brown rice, oats, and barley.
- **Nuts and Seeds:** Almonds, walnuts, flaxseeds, and chia seeds are not only high in healthy fats but also contain fiber, antioxidants, and minerals that help fight inflammation.
- **Healthy Fats:** Olive oil, especially extra-virgin olive oil, is rich in monounsaturated fats and antioxidants that have anti-inflammatory effects. Avocado is another excellent source of healthy fats and fiber.
- **Spices and Herbs:** Many spices and herbs, such as turmeric, ginger, garlic, and cinnamon, possess potent anti-inflammatory compounds. Turmeric, for instance, contains curcumin, a compound with strong anti-inflammatory and antioxidant properties.

The Role of Diet in Modulating Inflammation

The impact of diet on inflammation is multifaceted. Pro-inflammatory foods can induce an immune response, leading to increased production of inflammatory cytokines and markers like CRP. Over time, a diet high in these foods can contribute to the development and progression of chronic inflammatory diseases.

Conversely, anti-inflammatory foods can help to modulate the body's inflammatory response. They provide essential nutrients that support the immune system, reduce oxidative stress, and decrease the production of pro-inflammatory molecules. By altering the types of fats, carbohydrates, and overall nutrient density of the diet, individuals can significantly influence their inflammatory status.

Implementing an Anti-Inflammatory Diet

Transitioning to an anti-inflammatory diet involves more than just adding a few anti-inflammatory foods to your meals; it requires a holistic shift in dietary patterns. This includes:

- **Increasing intake of fruits, vegetables, whole grains, nuts, seeds, and healthy fats.**
- **Choosing lean protein sources and fatty fish rich in omega-3 fatty acids.**
- **Limiting consumption of processed foods, refined sugars, and carbohydrates.**
- **Balancing the intake of omega-6 and omega-3 fatty acids to improve the fatty acid ratio.**
- **Incorporating spices and herbs into meals for added flavor and anti-inflammatory benefits.**

By making these changes, individuals can create a dietary pattern that supports the body's natural ability to combat inflammation. This not only helps in managing existing inflammatory conditions but also plays a crucial role in preventing the onset of chronic diseases associated with inflammation."

# Long-term effects of chronic inflammation

"Chronic inflammation, a prolonged and persistent inflammatory response, can have far-reaching effects on the body, contributing to a range of health issues and chronic diseases. Unlike acute inflammation, which is a necessary and protective response to injury or infection, chronic inflammation can slowly damage the body's tissues, organs, and systems over time. This section outlines the long-term effects of chronic inflammation and its impact on overall health.

**Cardiovascular Diseases**

One of the most significant long-term effects of chronic inflammation is its impact on the cardiovascular system. Persistent inflammation can lead to the development of plaque in the arteries, a condition known as atherosclerosis. This plaque buildup can narrow and harden arteries, increasing the risk of heart attacks, strokes, and peripheral artery disease. Inflammation is also associated with hypertension (high blood pressure) and coronary artery disease, further elevating cardiovascular risk.

### Autoimmune Diseases

Chronic inflammation plays a central role in the development and progression of autoimmune diseases, where the immune system mistakenly attacks healthy cells and tissues. Conditions such as rheumatoid arthritis, lupus, and inflammatory bowel disease (IBD), including Crohn's disease and ulcerative colitis, are characterized by an overactive inflammatory response. This can lead to significant tissue damage, pain, and dysfunction in the affected organs.

### Metabolic Syndrome and Diabetes

Metabolic syndrome, a cluster of conditions including increased blood pressure, high blood sugar, excess body fat around the waist, and abnormal cholesterol levels, is closely linked to chronic inflammation. This syndrome significantly increases the risk of developing type 2 diabetes, heart disease, and stroke. Chronic inflammation is believed to contribute to insulin resistance, a key factor in the development of type 2 diabetes, further complicating metabolic health.

### Neurological Conditions

Emerging research suggests that chronic inflammation may also affect the brain, contributing to the development of neurological conditions and mental health disorders. Conditions such as Alzheimer's disease, Parkinson's disease, and multiple sclerosis have been linked to inflammatory processes. Additionally, chronic inflammation may influence the risk of depression, anxiety, and other mental health issues, highlighting the systemic impact of prolonged inflammation.

**Cancer**

Persistent inflammation has been identified as a significant risk factor for several types of cancer. Chronic inflammatory conditions can create an environment that promotes tumor growth, DNA damage, and cell mutation. Cancers of the colon, lung, and stomach, among others, have been associated with high levels of inflammation, underscoring the need for effective inflammation management.

**Digestive System Disorders**

The digestive tract is particularly susceptible to the effects of chronic inflammation. Conditions such as gastritis, peptic ulcers, and chronic hepatitis can arise from or be exacerbated by ongoing inflammatory responses. Inflammatory bowel disease, which includes Crohn's disease and ulcerative colitis, directly results from excessive inflammation in the gastrointestinal tract, leading to severe digestive issues, malnutrition, and increased colorectal cancer risk.

### Chronic Pain and Fatigue

Chronic inflammation can also lead to generalized symptoms such as chronic pain and fatigue. These symptoms can significantly impact quality of life, limiting daily activities and contributing to a cycle of physical deconditioning and further health decline.

## Managing Chronic Inflammation

Understanding the long-term effects of chronic inflammation underscores the importance of managing and reducing inflammatory responses through lifestyle changes, diet, and, when necessary, medical intervention. Adopting an anti-inflammatory diet, engaging in regular physical activity, managing stress, and ensuring adequate sleep is all critical strategies in mitigating the adverse effects of chronic inflammation."

*Chapter 2*

# The 10 Proven Secrets to a Transformative Anti-Inflammatory Diet

## Secret 1: Incorporate Anti-Inflammatory Superfoods

"The foundation of an anti-inflammatory diet is built on superfoods known for their potent anti-inflammatory properties. These foods are rich in antioxidants, vitamins, and minerals that help reduce inflammation throughout the body. Incorporating a variety of these superfoods into your diet can significantly enhance your health and protect against chronic diseases.

- **List of Superfoods:** Berries, dark leafy greens (such as spinach and kale), beets, broccoli, nuts (like almonds and walnuts), seeds (such as flaxseeds and chia seeds), olive oil, and fatty fish (like salmon and mackerel) are all excellent choices. These foods are not only high in nutrients but also contain powerful antioxidants that fight inflammation.

- **Benefits and Nutritional Information:** Superfoods offer a wide range of health benefits beyond inflammation reduction. They can improve heart health, enhance brain function, and support immune system health. For instance, berries are rich in flavonoids, which have been shown to reduce the risk of heart disease."

## Secret 2: Focus on Omega-3 Fatty Acids

"Omega-3 fatty acids are crucial for reducing inflammation and are essential for overall health. They are particularly effective in combating inflammation associated with chronic diseases.

- **Sources of Omega-3s:** The best sources include fatty fish like salmon, mackerel, and sardines, as well as plant-based sources like flaxseeds, chia seeds, and walnuts.

- **Omega-3s' Role in Reducing Inflammation:** These fatty acids produce resolvins and protectins, which have anti-inflammatory effects. They can decrease the production of molecules and substances linked to inflammation, such as eicosanoids and cytokines."

## Secret 3: Hydrate and Choose Anti-Inflammatory Drinks

"Hydration is a key to maintaining optimal health and combating inflammation. The fluids you choose can either contribute to or reduce inflammation.

- **Importance of Hydration:** Proper hydration helps flush toxins from the body, which can reduce inflammation. It also ensures that nutrients are efficiently transported to cells, aiding in their optimal function.

- **Recipes for Anti-Inflammatory Drinks:** Green tea, known for its epigallocatechin gallate (EGCG) content, and turmeric tea, rich in curcumin, are powerful anti-inflammatory beverages. Incorporating these drinks into your daily routine can provide a significant boost to your anti-inflammatory efforts."

## Secret 4: Eliminate or Reduce Inflammatory Foods

"Reducing the intake of foods known to cause inflammation is crucial for managing and preventing chronic inflammation.

- **Foods to Avoid:** Processed foods, refined sugars, and trans fats are among the top contributors to inflammation. Red meat and processed meats are also known to promote inflammation.

- **Tips for Cutting Out Processed Foods:** Focus on whole, unprocessed foods and make gradual changes to your diet. Reading labels to avoid products with high sugar content or unhealthy fats can also make a significant difference."

## Secret 5: Optimize Gut Health for Better Immunity

"The health of your gut plays a critical role in inflammation and overall health due to its direct link to the immune system.

- **Connection Between Gut Health and Inflammation:** A healthy gut microbiome can prevent the entrance of harmful pathogens that trigger inflammation. An imbalance, however, can lead to increased permeability ("leaky gut"), allowing toxins to enter the bloodstream and cause inflammation.

- **Probiotic and Prebiotic Foods:** Foods rich in probiotics (like yogurt, kefir, and sauerkraut) and prebiotics (such as garlic, onions, and bananas) support a healthy gut microbiome, reducing inflammation."

# Secret 6: Spice Up Your Diet with Anti-Inflammatory Spices

"Spices and herbs are not only great for adding flavor to dishes but also possess powerful anti-inflammatory properties.

- **Healing Spices and Herbs:** Turmeric, ginger, garlic, and cinnamon are among the top spices known for their anti-inflammatory effects. Curcumin in turmeric, in particular, is highly effective in reducing inflammation.

- **How to Incorporate Them into Meals:** Add these spices to soups, stews, smoothies, and teas to enhance flavor and health benefits. Turmeric can be combined with black pepper to increase its absorption."

# Secret 7: Embrace Healthy Fats

"Understanding and choosing healthy fats over unhealthy ones is crucial for reducing inflammation.

- **Differentiating Healthy and Unhealthy Fats:** Monounsaturated and polyunsaturated fats, found in foods like avocados, nuts, and seeds, as well as olive oil, are beneficial. In contrast, saturated and trans fats found in processed foods should be limited.

- **Recipes Highlighting Healthy Fats:** Incorporating avocado into salads, using olive oil as a dressing, and adding nuts and seeds to dishes are great ways to include healthy fats in your diet."

## Secret 8: Adapt Portion Control and Mindful Eating

"Eating the right amount of food and being mindful about eating can significantly impact inflammation and overall health.

- **Strategies for Portion Control:** Use smaller plates, listen to hunger cues, and avoid eating directly from large packages. This can help prevent overeating, which is linked to increased inflammation.
- **Benefits of Mindful Eating:** Being mindful of what and how much you eat can improve digestion, reduce stress eating, and support a healthy inflammatory response."

## Secret 9: Incorporate Regular Detoxification

"Regularly consuming foods that support the body's natural detox processes can help reduce inflammation.

- **Natural Detox Foods and Their Benefits:** Foods like leafy greens, beets, and citrus fruits support liver health and promote the elimination of toxins. This can lower the body's inflammatory response.

- **Simple Detox Meal Ideas:** Incorporating a daily green smoothie or a salad rich in detoxifying vegetables can be an easy and delicious way to support your body's detoxification processes."

## Secret 10: Combine Diet with Lifestyle Changes

"Last but not least, combining dietary changes with lifestyle modifications can maximize the anti-inflammatory benefits.

- **Exercise and Its Anti-Inflammatory Effects:** Regular physical activity can reduce inflammation throughout the body by improving circulation and helping to manage weight.

- **Stress Reduction Techniques and Sleep's Role in Inflammation:** Managing stress through techniques like meditation and ensuring adequate sleep each night are essential for controlling inflammation. Chronic stress and lack of sleep can both increase inflammation.

By integrating these ten secrets into your life, you can significantly reduce inflammation and embark on a path toward a healthier, more vibrant lifestyle. This chapter not only serves as a guide to adopting an anti-inflammatory diet but also emphasizes the importance of a holistic approach to health that includes both dietary and lifestyle factors."

*Chapter 3*

# Beginner-Friendly Recipes

## Breakfasts

### 1. Golden Turmeric and Ginger Smoothie

**"Prep Time:** 5 minutes | **Cook Time:** 0 minutes | **Servings:** 2

**Ingredients:**

- 1 ripe banana
- 1 inch fresh ginger, peeled
- 1/2 teaspoon ground turmeric
- 1 tablespoon honey (optional)
- 1 cup unsweetened almond milk
- Ice cubes

**Directions:**

1. Place the banana, ginger, turmeric, honey (if using), and almond milk in a blender.
2. Add a handful of ice cubes.
3. Blend on high speed until smooth and creamy.

4. Taste and adjust sweetness, adding more honey if desired.

5. Pour into glasses and serve immediately.

   **Nutritional Information:** (approximation)

   - Calories: 120
   - Protein: 1.5g
   - Fat: 1.5g
   - Carbohydrates: 28g
   - Fiber: 3g

2. Omega-3 Rich Chia Pudding

   **Prep Time:** 8 hours (overnight) | **Cook Time:** 0 minutes | **Servings:** 2

   **Ingredients:**

   - 1/4 cup chia seeds
   - 1 cup unsweetened almond milk
   - 1/2 teaspoon vanilla extract
   - 1 tablespoon maple syrup
   - 1/2 cup mixed berries (fresh or frozen)
   - 1 tablespoon flaxseeds

   **Directions:**

1. In a medium bowl, combine chia seeds, almond milk, vanilla extract, and maple syrup. Stir well to combine.
2. Cover and refrigerate overnight or at least 8 hours, until it has a pudding-like consistency.
3. Before serving, stir the pudding to break any clumps.
4. Serve topped with mixed berries and a sprinkle of flaxseeds.

**Nutritional Information:** (approximation)

- Calories: 180
- Protein: 4g
- Fat: 9g
- Carbohydrates: 20g
- Fiber: 8g

### 3. Spinach and Avocado Breakfast Salad

**Prep Time:** 10 minutes | **Cook Time:** 5 minutes | **Servings:** 2

**Ingredients:**

- 2 cups baby spinach
- 1 ripe avocado, sliced
- 1/4 cup walnuts, roughly chopped
- 2 eggs

- 2 tablespoons extra virgin olive oil
- 1 tablespoon lemon juice
- Salt and pepper, to taste

**Directions:**

1. Bring a small pot of water to a boil. Gently add the eggs and cook for 6-7 minutes for soft-boiled eggs. Remove and place in cold water to cool before peeling.
2. In a large bowl, combine the spinach, avocado slices, and chopped walnuts.
3. In a small bowl, whisk together the olive oil, lemon juice, salt, and pepper.
4. Peel and halve the eggs.
5. Drizzle the dressing over the salad and gently toss to combine.
6. Top the salad with the soft-boiled eggs and serve immediately.

**Nutritional Information:** (approximation)

- Calories: 320
- Protein: 8g
- Fat: 27g
- Carbohydrates: 14g
- Fiber: 7g

## 4. Sweet Potato and Kale Hash

**Prep Time:** 10 minutes | **Cook Time:** 20 minutes | **Servings:** 2

**Ingredients:**

- 1 large sweet potato, peeled and diced
- 2 cups kale, chopped
- 1 small onion, diced
- 1 clove garlic, minced
- 2 tablespoons olive oil
- 2 eggs
- Salt and pepper, to taste

**Directions:**

1. Heat the olive oil in a large skillet over medium heat. Add the diced sweet potato and onion. Cook, stirring occasionally, until the sweet potatoes are tender, about 10 minutes.

2. Add the minced garlic and chopped kale to the skillet. Cook until the kale is wilted and the garlic is fragrant, about 3-4 minutes.

3. Create two wells in the hash and crack an egg into each well. Cover the skillet and cook until the eggs are set to your liking, about 4-5 minutes for soft yolks.

4. Season with salt and pepper to taste. Serve the hash with the eggs on top.

**Nutritional Information:** (approximation)

- Calories: 300
- Protein: 10g
- Fat: 18g
- Carbohydrates: 24g
- Fiber: 4g

## 5. Anti-Inflammatory Overnight Oats

**Prep Time:** 8 hours (overnight) | **Cook Time:** 0 minutes | **Servings:** 2

**Ingredients:**

- 1 cup rolled oats
- 1 cup unsweetened almond milk
- 1/2 teaspoon ground turmeric
- 1/2 teaspoon ground cinnamon
- 1 apple, cored and diced
- 1 tablespoon almond butter
- 1 tablespoon honey or maple syrup (optional)

**Directions:**

1. In a medium bowl, mix together the oats, almond milk, turmeric, and cinnamon. Stir in the diced apple.
2. Cover and refrigerate overnight.

3. In the morning, stir the oats well. If the mixture is too thick, add a little more almond milk to reach your desired consistency.
4. Serve the oats topped with a dollop of almond butter and a drizzle of honey or maple syrup, if using.

**Nutritional Information:** (approximation)

- Calories: 250
- Protein: 6g
- Fat: 7g
- Carbohydrates: 40g
- Fiber: 6g

6. Quinoa Breakfast Bowl with Mixed Berries

    **Prep Time:** 5 minutes | **Cook Time:** 15 minutes | **Servings:** 2

    **Ingredients:**

- 1/2 cup quinoa, rinsed
- 1 cup water
- 1/2 cup mixed berries (such as strawberries, blueberries, raspberries)
- 2 tablespoons almond butter
- 1 tablespoon hemp seeds

**Directions:**

1. In a small saucepan, combine quinoa and water. Bring to a boil over high heat.
2. Reduce heat to low, cover, and simmer for 15 minutes, or until quinoa is fluffy and water is absorbed.
3. Remove from heat and let it sit, covered, for 5 minutes. Fluff with a fork.
4. Divide the cooked quinoa into bowls. Top with mixed berries, a dollop of almond butter, and a sprinkle of hemp seeds.
5. Serve warm, adding a splash of almond milk if desired.

**Nutritional Information:** (approximation)

- Calories: 280
- Protein: 9g
- Fat: 10g
- Carbohydrates: 40g
- Fiber: 6g

## 7. Broccoli and Red Pepper Frittata

**Prep Time:** 10 minutes | **Cook Time:** 20 minutes | **Servings:** 4

**Ingredients:**

- 6 eggs

- 1 cup broccoli florets
- 1 red bell pepper, diced
- 1/2 teaspoon turmeric
- Salt and pepper, to taste
- 1 tablespoon olive oil

**Directions:**

1. Preheat the oven to 375°F (190°C).
2. In a bowl, beat the eggs with turmeric, salt, and pepper.
3. Heat olive oil in an oven-safe skillet over medium heat. Add broccoli and red pepper, sautéing until slightly softened, about 5 minutes.
4. Pour the beaten eggs over the vegetables, tilting the pan to distribute them evenly.
5. Cook without stirring for about 2 minutes, until the edges start to set.
6. Transfer the skillet to the oven and bake for 15-18 minutes, or until the frittata is set and lightly golden on top.
7. Let cool for a few minutes before slicing and serving.

**Nutritional Information:** (approximation)

- Calories: 160
- Protein: 11g

- Fat: 11g
- Carbohydrates: 5g
- Fiber: 1g

## 8. Salmon Avocado Toast

**Prep Time:** 5 minutes | **Cook Time:** 0 minutes | **Servings:** 2

**Ingredients:**

- 2 slices whole-grain bread
- 1 ripe avocado
- 4 ounces smoked salmon
- 1 teaspoon lemon juice
- Salt and pepper, to taste
- 1 tablespoon chia seeds

**Directions:**

1. Toast the whole-grain bread slices until golden and crispy.
2. In a small bowl, mash the avocado with lemon juice, salt, and pepper.
3. Spread the mashed avocado evenly over the toasted bread slices.
4. Top each slice with smoked salmon.
5. Sprinkle chia seeds over the top for an extra nutrient boost.

6. Serve immediately, enjoying the blend of flavors and textures.

   **Nutritional Information:** (approximation)

- Calories: 300
- Protein: 15g
- Fat: 20g
- Carbohydrates: 20g
- Fiber: 7g

## 9. Beetroot and Ginger Detox Juice

**Prep Time:** 10 minutes | **Cook Time:** 0 minutes | **Servings:** 2

**Ingredients:**

- 1 medium beetroot, peeled and chopped
- 1 inch ginger, peeled
- 2 carrots, peeled and chopped
- 1 apple, cored and chopped
- 1/2 cup water (optional, for easier blending)

**Directions:**

1. Place the beetroot, ginger, carrots, and apple in a juicer.
2. Process until smooth. If using a blender, add a little water to help blend the ingredients, then strain through a fine mesh sieve or cheesecloth.

3. Pour the juice into glasses and drink immediately for the best nutrient intake.

   **Nutritional Information:** (approximation)

- Calories: 100
- Protein: 2g
- Fat: 0.5g
- Carbohydrates: 24g
- Fiber: 6g

## 10. Blueberry and Walnut Steel-Cut Oats

**Prep Time:** 5 minutes | **Cook Time:** 25 minutes | **Servings:** 2

**Ingredients:**

- 1/2 cup steel-cut oats
- 2 cups water
- Pinch of salt
- 1/2 cup blueberries
- 1/4 cup walnuts, chopped
- 1/2 teaspoon ground cinnamon

**Directions:**

1. In a medium saucepan, bring water to a boil. Add steel-cut oats and a pinch of salt.

2. Reduce heat to low, cover, and simmer for 20-25 minutes, or until oats are tender and water is absorbed.
3. Remove from heat and let sit for 5 minutes. Stir in the ground cinnamon.
4. Serve the oats topped with blueberries and chopped walnuts.

**Nutritional Information:** (approximation)

- Calories: 220
- Protein: 6g
- Fat: 10g
- Carbohydrates: 30g
- Fiber: 5g

## 11. Green Tea Infused Chia Breakfast Pudding

**Prep Time:** 8 hours (overnight) | **Cook Time:** 0 minutes | **Servings:** 2

**Ingredients:**

- 1/4 cup chia seeds
- 1 cup brewed green tea, cooled
- 1/2 mango, peeled and pureed
- 1 tablespoon coconut flakes

**Directions:**

1. In a medium bowl, mix together the chia seeds and cooled green tea. Cover and refrigerate overnight.
2. In the morning, stir the pudding to ensure it has a consistent texture.
3. Layer the chia pudding with mango puree in serving glasses.
4. Top with coconut flakes before serving.

**Nutritional Information:** (approximation)

- Calories: 150
- Protein: 3g
- Fat: 7g
- Carbohydrates: 19g
- Fiber: 9g

## 12. Zucchini and Basil Breakfast Muffins

**Prep Time:** 15 minutes | **Cook Time:** 20 minutes | **Servings:** 12 muffins

**Ingredients:**

- 2 cups almond flour
- 1 teaspoon baking powder
- 1/4 teaspoon salt
- 3 eggs

- 1/4 cup olive oil
- 1 cup zucchini, grated and excess moisture squeezed out
- 1/4 cup fresh basil, chopped

**Directions:**

1. Preheat the oven to 350°F (175°C). Line a muffin tin with paper liners or grease with olive oil.
2. In a large bowl, combine almond flour, baking powder, and salt.
3. In another bowl, whisk together the eggs and olive oil. Stir in the grated zucchini and chopped basil.
4. Add the wet ingredients to the dry ingredients, stirring until just combined.
5. Divide the batter evenly among the muffin cups.
6. Bake for 20-25 minutes, or until a toothpick inserted into the center of a muffin comes out clean.
7. Let the muffins cool in the pan for 5 minutes before transferring to a wire rack to cool completely.

**Nutritional Information:** (approximation)

- Calories: 180
- Protein: 6g

- Fat: 15g
- Carbohydrates: 8g
- Fiber: 3g"

# Lunches

### 13. Mediterranean Quinoa Salad

"**Prep Time:** 15 minutes | **Cook Time:** 20 minutes | **Servings:** 4

**Ingredients:**

- 1 cup quinoa
- 2 cups water
- 1 cucumber, diced
- 1 cup cherry tomatoes, halved
- 1/2 cup Kalamata olives, pitted and halved
- 1/4 red onion, thinly sliced
- 1/2 cup feta cheese, crumbled
- 1/4 cup extra virgin olive oil
- Juice of 1 lemon
- Salt and pepper, to taste

**Directions:**

1. Rinse quinoa under cold water. In a medium saucepan, bring 2 cups of water to a boil. Add quinoa, reduce heat to low, cover, and simmer

for 15 minutes or until water is absorbed. Fluff with a fork and let cool.

2. In a large bowl, combine cooled quinoa, cucumber, cherry tomatoes, Kalamata olives, red onion, and feta cheese.

3. In a small bowl, whisk together olive oil, lemon juice, salt, and pepper. Pour over the salad and toss to combine.

4. Serve chilled or at room temperature.

**Nutritional Information:** (approximation)

- Calories: 320
- Protein: 8g
- Fat: 18g
- Carbohydrates: 30g
- Fiber: 4g

### 14. Turmeric Chicken Wraps

**Prep Time:** 20 minutes (plus marination time) | **Cook Time:** 10 minutes | **Servings:** 4

**Ingredients:**

- 2 chicken breasts, thinly sliced
- 1 teaspoon ground turmeric
- 1 garlic clove, minced
- 1 inch ginger, minced

- 2 tablespoons olive oil
- 4 whole wheat wraps
- 1 avocado, sliced
- 2 cups mixed greens
- Salt and pepper, to taste

**Directions:**

1. In a bowl, combine chicken slices, turmeric, garlic, ginger, 1 tablespoon olive oil, salt, and pepper. Marinate for at least 30 minutes in the refrigerator.
2. Heat the remaining olive oil in a pan over medium heat. Add the chicken and cook for 5-7 minutes, or until fully cooked.
3. Warm the wraps according to package instructions.
4. Assemble the wraps by laying out the mixed greens, cooked chicken, and avocado slices on each wrap.
5. Roll up the wraps, cut in half, and serve.

**Nutritional Information:** (approximation)

- Calories: 350
- Protein: 25g
- Fat: 15g
- Carbohydrates: 30g
- Fiber: 5g

## 15. Sweet Potato and Black Bean Buddha Bowl

**Prep Time:** 10 minutes | **Cook Time:** 25 minutes | **Servings:** 4

**Ingredients:**
- 2 medium sweet potatoes, peeled and cubed
- 1 tablespoon olive oil
- Salt and pepper, to taste
- 1 can (15 oz) black beans, rinsed and drained
- 4 cups spinach
- 1 avocado, sliced
- 1/4 cup seeds (pumpkin or sunflower)
- For the lime tahini dressing:
    - 1/4 cup tahini
    - Juice of 1 lime
    - 2 tablespoons water
    - Salt, to taste

**Directions:**
1. Preheat oven to 400°F (200°C). Toss sweet potatoes with olive oil, salt, and pepper. Spread on a baking sheet and roast for 20-25 minutes, until tender.

2. Prepare the lime tahini dressing by whisking together tahini, lime juice, water, and salt until smooth.

3. Assemble the Buddha bowls by dividing the spinach, roasted sweet potatoes, black beans, and avocado slices among 4 bowls.

4. Drizzle with lime tahini dressing and sprinkle with seeds.

5. Serve immediately.

**Nutritional Information:** (approximation)

- Calories: 380
- Protein: 12g
- Fat: 18g
- Carbohydrates: 45g
- Fiber: 12g

## 16. Zesty Salmon Salad

**Prep Time:** 15 minutes | **Cook Time:** 0 minutes | **Servings:** 2

**Ingredients:**

- 2 cups mixed greens (such as arugula and spinach)
- 1 avocado, sliced
- 2 small oranges, peeled and segmented

- 8 oz cooked salmon, flaked
- For the dressing:
    - 2 tablespoons olive oil
    - Juice of 1 lemon
    - 1 teaspoon honey
    - Salt and pepper, to taste

**Directions:**

1. In a large bowl, combine mixed greens, avocado slices, and orange segments.
2. Gently fold in the flaked salmon, being careful not to break the pieces too much.
3. In a small bowl, whisk together olive oil, lemon juice, honey, salt, and pepper to create the dressing.
4. Drizzle the dressing over the salad and toss gently to combine.
5. Divide the salad between two plates and serve immediately.

**Nutritional Information:** (approximation)

- Calories: 450
- Protein: 25g
- Fat: 30g
- Carbohydrates: 20g
- Fiber: 7g

## 17. Butternut Squash Soup

**Prep Time:** 10 minutes | **Cook Time:** 30 minutes | **Servings:** 4

**Ingredients:**

- 1 medium butternut squash, peeled, seeded, and cubed
- 1 tablespoon olive oil
- 1 small onion, chopped
- 1 clove garlic, minced
- 4 cups vegetable broth
- 1/2 teaspoon ground ginger
- 1/4 teaspoon ground nutmeg
- Salt and pepper, to taste

**Directions:**

1. In a large pot, heat olive oil over medium heat. Add onion and garlic, sautéing until soft, about 5 minutes.
2. Add the cubed butternut squash and cook for another 5 minutes.
3. Pour in the vegetable broth, and add ginger, nutmeg, salt, and pepper. Bring to a boil.
4. Reduce heat and simmer until squash is tender, about 20 minutes.

5. Use an immersion blender to puree the soup until smooth (or transfer to a blender in batches).
6. Serve hot, with a side of whole-grain bread if desired.

**Nutritional Information:** (approximation)

- Calories: 180
- Protein: 3g
- Fat: 5g
- Carbohydrates: 33g
- Fiber: 5g

## 18. Kale and White Bean Stew

**Prep Time:** 10 minutes | **Cook Time:** 30 minutes | **Servings:** 4

**Ingredients:**

- 1 tablespoon olive oil
- 1 onion, diced
- 2 carrots, diced
- 2 cloves garlic, minced
- 4 cups kale, chopped
- 1 can (15 oz) white beans, rinsed and drained
- 1 can (14.5 oz) diced tomatoes, undrained

- 4 cups vegetable broth
- 1 teaspoon rosemary, minced
- 1 teaspoon thyme
- Salt and pepper, to taste

**Directions:**

1. Heat olive oil in a large pot over medium heat. Add onion, carrots, and garlic; sauté until vegetables are soft, about 5 minutes.
2. Add kale, and cook until it starts to wilt, about 3 minutes.
3. Stir in white beans, diced tomatoes with their juice, vegetable broth, rosemary, thyme, salt, and pepper.
4. Bring to a boil, then reduce heat and simmer for 20 minutes.
5. Taste and adjust seasoning if necessary. Serve hot.

**Nutritional Information:** (approximation)

- Calories: 220
- Protein: 10g
- Fat: 4g
- Carbohydrates: 37g
- Fiber: 9g

## 19. Avocado and Egg Toast

**Prep Time:** 5 minutes | **Cook Time:** 5 minutes | **Servings:** 2

**Ingredients:**

- 2 slices of whole-grain bread
- 1 ripe avocado
- 2 eggs
- Chili flakes, to taste
- Salt and pepper, to taste

**Directions:**

1. Toast the bread slices to your liking.
2. Meanwhile, poach the eggs. Bring a pot of water to a simmer, gently crack the eggs into the water, and cook for 3-4 minutes for soft yolks or longer for firmer yolks. Remove with a slotted spoon.
3. Mash the avocado with a fork and season with salt and pepper. Spread evenly over the toasted bread.
4. Top each slice with a poached egg. Sprinkle with chili flakes for a bit of heat.
5. Serve immediately, enjoying the combination of creamy avocado and rich, runny egg.

**Nutritional Information:** (approximation)

- Calories: 350

- Protein: 12g
- Fat: 20g
- Carbohydrates: 30g
- Fiber: 8g

## 20. Cauliflower Rice Stir-Fry

**Prep Time:** 10 minutes | **Cook Time:** 10 minutes | **Servings:** 2

**Ingredients:**

- 1 head cauliflower, grated into rice-sized pieces
- 1 tablespoon olive oil
- 2 cups mixed vegetables (e.g., carrots, peas, bell peppers), diced
- 2 cloves garlic, minced
- 1 inch ginger, minced
- 2 tablespoons tamari or soy sauce
- 1 tablespoon sesame seeds

**Directions:**

1. Heat olive oil in a large pan over medium heat. Add garlic and ginger, sautéing until fragrant, about 1 minute.

2. Increase the heat to medium-high and add the mixed vegetables. Stir-fry for 3-4 minutes until they start to soften.
3. Add the cauliflower rice and tamari or soy sauce. Cook, stirring frequently, for 5-6 minutes, until the vegetables are tender and the cauliflower is heated through.
4. Sprinkle with sesame seeds before serving.

**Nutritional Information:** (approximation)

- Calories: 200
- Protein: 6g
- Fat: 10g
- Carbohydrates: 24g
- Fiber: 8g

## 21. Roasted Chickpea and Broccoli Bowl

**Prep Time:** 10 minutes | **Cook Time:** 20 minutes | **Servings:** 2

**Ingredients:**

- 1 can (15 oz) chickpeas, drained, rinsed, and dried
- 2 cups broccoli florets
- 1 tablespoon olive oil
- Salt and pepper, to taste

- 1 cup cooked quinoa
- For the tahini sauce:
    - 2 tablespoons tahini
    - 1 tablespoon lemon juice
    - 1 clove garlic, minced
    - Water, as needed to thin

**Directions:**

1. Preheat the oven to 400°F (200°C). Toss chickpeas and broccoli with olive oil, salt, and pepper. Spread on a baking sheet.
2. Roast for 20 minutes, or until chickpeas are crispy and broccoli is tender.
3. While the chickpeas and broccoli roast, prepare the tahini sauce by whisking together tahini, lemon juice, garlic, and enough water to achieve a pourable consistency.
4. Divide the cooked quinoa between bowls, top with roasted chickpeas and broccoli, and drizzle with tahini sauce.

**Nutritional Information:** (approximation)

- Calories: 400
- Protein: 15g
- Fat: 20g
- Carbohydrates: 45g
- Fiber: 10g

## 22. Beet and Goat Cheese Arugula Salad

**Prep Time:** 10 minutes | **Cook Time:** 0 minutes | **Servings:** 2

**Ingredients:**

- 4 cups arugula
- 2 medium beets, roasted, peeled, and sliced
- 1/4 cup goat cheese, crumbled
- 1/4 cup walnuts, toasted
- 2 tablespoons balsamic reduction

**Directions:**

1. In a large salad bowl, combine arugula, sliced beets, goat cheese, and walnuts.
2. Drizzle with balsamic reduction just before serving.
3. Toss lightly to combine. Serve immediately for a fresh, flavorful salad.

**Nutritional Information:** (approximation)

- Calories: 250
- Protein: 8g
- Fat: 18g
- Carbohydrates: 16g

## 23. Lentil and Vegetable Curry

**Prep Time:** 10 minutes | **Cook Time:** 30 minutes | **Servings:** 4

**Ingredients:**

- 1 cup red lentils, rinsed
- 1 sweet potato, peeled and cubed
- 2 cups spinach, roughly chopped
- 1 can (14 oz) coconut milk
- 1 onion, diced
- 2 garlic cloves, minced
- 1 tablespoon curry powder
- 1 teaspoon turmeric
- 2 tablespoons olive oil
- Salt to taste
- 2 cups water or vegetable broth
- Cooked brown rice, for serving

**Directions:**

1. Heat olive oil in a large pot over medium heat. Add the diced onion and minced garlic, sautéing until soft and translucent.
2. Stir in curry powder and turmeric, cooking for another minute until fragrant.
3. Add the rinsed lentils, cubed sweet potato, and water or vegetable broth. Bring to a boil.

4. Reduce heat, cover, and simmer for about 20 minutes, or until lentils are soft and sweet potatoes are tender.
5. Stir in coconut milk and chopped spinach, cooking for an additional 5 minutes. Season with salt to taste.
6. Serve the curry over cooked brown rice.

   **Nutritional Information:** (approximation)
- Calories: 400
- Protein: 18g
- Fat: 18g
- Carbohydrates: 50g
- Fiber: 15g

## 24. Grilled Vegetable and Hummus Flatbread

**Prep Time:** 15 minutes | **Cook Time:** 10 minutes | **Servings:** 4

**Ingredients:**
- 4 whole-grain flatbreads
- 1 zucchini, sliced into thin rounds
- 1 red bell pepper, sliced into strips
- 1 red onion, sliced into rings
- 1 cup hummus

- 2 tablespoons olive oil
- Salt and pepper, to taste
- Optional toppings: fresh basil, cherry tomatoes, balsamic glaze

**Directions:**

1. Preheat your grill or grill pan over medium heat.
2. Toss the zucchini, bell pepper, and onion with olive oil, salt, and pepper.
3. Grill the vegetables for about 5-7 minutes, turning occasionally, until they are tender and have grill marks.
4. Spread hummus evenly over each flatbread.
5. Arrange the grilled vegetables on top of the hummus.
6. If using, add fresh basil, cherry tomatoes, and a drizzle of balsamic glaze for extra flavor.
7. Serve immediately, cut into slices.

**Nutritional Information:** (approximation)

- Calories: 350
- Protein: 12g
- Fat: 15g
- Carbohydrates: 45g
- Fiber: 8g"

# Dinners

### 25. Ginger-Soy Glazed Salmon

"**Prep Time:** 10 minutes | **Cook Time:** 20 minutes | **Servings:** 4

**Ingredients:**

- 4 salmon fillets (6 ounces each)
- 2 tablespoons soy sauce
- 1 tablespoon honey
- 1 tablespoon fresh ginger, grated
- 1 garlic clove, minced
- 1 tablespoon olive oil
- 2 cups broccoli florets
- Salt and pepper, to taste

**Directions:**

1. Preheat the oven to 375°F (190°C). Line a baking sheet with parchment paper.
2. In a small bowl, whisk together soy sauce, honey, ginger, and garlic.
3. Place salmon fillets on the prepared baking sheet. Brush each fillet with the soy-ginger glaze.
4. Toss broccoli florets with olive oil, salt, and pepper. Scatter around the salmon on the baking sheet.

5. Bake for 18-20 minutes, or until salmon is opaque and flakes easily with a fork, and broccoli is tender.
6. Serve the glazed salmon with steamed broccoli on the side.

**Nutritional Information:** (approximation)
- Calories: 300
- Protein: 23g
- Fat: 15g
- Carbohydrates: 10g
- Fiber: 2g

## 26. Turmeric Roasted Chicken and Vegetables

**Prep Time:** 15 minutes | **Cook Time:** 40 minutes | **Servings:** 4

**Ingredients:**
- 4 chicken thighs, bone-in and skin-on
- 2 carrots, sliced
- 1 bell pepper, cut into strips
- 1 zucchini, sliced
- 2 tablespoons olive oil
- 1 teaspoon ground turmeric
- 2 garlic cloves, minced

- Salt and pepper, to taste

**Directions:**

1. Preheat the oven to 400°F (200°C). Line a large baking tray with parchment paper.
2. In a large bowl, combine olive oil, turmeric, garlic, salt, and pepper.
3. Add chicken thighs and vegetables to the bowl. Toss well to coat everything in the turmeric mixture.
4. Arrange the chicken and vegetables in a single layer on the prepared baking tray.
5. Roast for 35-40 minutes, or until the chicken is cooked through and vegetables are tender.
6. Serve hot, with a side of quinoa or brown rice if desired.

**Nutritional Information:** (approximation)

- Calories: 350
- Protein: 24g
- Fat: 22g
- Carbohydrates: 12g
- Fiber: 3g

## 27. Spicy Sweet Potato and Black Bean Chili

**Prep Time:** 10 minutes | **Cook Time:** 30 minutes | **Servings:** 4

**Ingredients:**

- 2 tablespoons olive oil
- 1 onion, diced
- 2 garlic cloves, minced
- 2 sweet potatoes, peeled and cubed
- 1 can (15 oz) black beans, rinsed and drained
- 1 can (14.5 oz) diced tomatoes
- 2 cups vegetable broth
- 1 tablespoon chili powder
- 1 teaspoon cumin
- Salt and pepper, to taste
- Optional toppings: avocado, cilantro, lime wedges

**Directions:**

1. Heat olive oil in a large pot over medium heat. Add onion and garlic; sauté until soft, about 5 minutes.
2. Add sweet potatoes, black beans, diced tomatoes (with juice), vegetable broth, chili powder, cumin, salt, and pepper to the pot.

3. Bring to a boil, then reduce heat to low and simmer, uncovered, for 25-30 minutes, or until sweet potatoes are tender.

4. Serve hot, garnished with avocado, cilantro, and lime wedges if desired.

**Nutritional Information:** (approximation)

- Calories: 250
- Protein: 8g
- Fat: 7g
- Carbohydrates: 40g
- Fiber: 10g

## 28. Lemon Garlic Shrimp with Zucchini Noodles

**Prep Time:** 10 minutes | **Cook Time:** 10 minutes | **Servings:** 4

**Ingredients:**

- 1 pound (450g) shrimp, peeled and deveined
- 2 tablespoons olive oil
- 3 garlic cloves, minced
- Juice of 1 lemon
- 4 zucchinis, spiralized into noodles
- Salt and pepper, to taste
- Red pepper flakes, optional

**Directions:**

1. Heat 1 tablespoon of olive oil in a large skillet over medium heat. Add garlic and sauté for 1 minute until fragrant.
2. Add shrimp to the skillet. Season with salt, pepper, and red pepper flakes if using. Cook for 2-3 minutes per side, or until shrimp are pink and opaque.
3. Remove shrimp from the skillet and set aside. In the same skillet, add the remaining olive oil and zucchini noodles. Sauté for 2-3 minutes, until noodles are tender.
4. Return shrimp to the skillet. Add lemon juice and toss everything together to heat through.
5. Serve immediately, garnished with lemon wedges if desired.

**Nutritional Information:** (approximation)

- Calories: 220
- Protein: 25g
- Fat: 10g
- Carbohydrates: 8g
- Fiber: 2g

## 29. Stuffed Bell Peppers with Quinoa and Ground Turkey

**Prep Time:** 15 minutes | **Cook Time:** 30 minutes | **Servings:** 4

**Ingredients:**

- 4 bell peppers, tops cut off and seeds removed
- 1 cup quinoa, cooked
- 1 pound (450g) ground turkey
- 1 can (14.5 oz) diced tomatoes, drained
- 1 onion, diced
- 2 cloves garlic, minced
- 1 teaspoon cumin
- 1 teaspoon paprika
- 1/2 cup shredded cheese (optional)
- Salt and pepper, to taste
- Olive oil

**Directions:**

1. Preheat oven to 375°F (190°C). Drizzle the inside of the bell peppers with olive oil and season with salt and pepper. Place them in a baking dish.
2. Heat a skillet over medium heat. Add a splash of olive oil, diced onion, and minced garlic. Sauté until softened, about 5 minutes.

3. Add ground turkey to the skillet. Cook, breaking it apart with a spoon, until no longer pink.

4. Stir in cooked quinoa, diced tomatoes, cumin, paprika, salt, and pepper. Cook for another 5 minutes.

5. Spoon the mixture into the prepared bell peppers. Top with shredded cheese if using.

6. Bake for 20-25 minutes, or until peppers are tender and cheese is melted.

7. Serve hot.

**Nutritional Information:** (approximation)

- Calories: 350
- Protein: 26g
- Fat: 12g
- Carbohydrates: 35g
- Fiber: 6g

## 30. Miso Soup with Tofu and Seaweed

**Prep Time:** 5 minutes | **Cook Time:** 10 minutes | **Servings:** 4

**Ingredients:**

- 4 cups water

- 2 tablespoons miso paste
- 1 block silken tofu, cubed
- 1/4 cup dried seaweed, rehydrated
- 2 green onions, thinly sliced

**Directions:**

1. In a pot, bring water to a simmer. Do not boil.
2. Place miso paste in a small bowl. Add a little hot water and whisk until smooth.
3. Add the miso mixture back into the pot with simmering water. Stir well.
4. Add cubed tofu and rehydrated seaweed to the pot. Warm through for about 3 minutes, ensuring not to boil.
5. Serve the soup in bowls, garnished with sliced green onions.

**Nutritional Information:** (approximation)

- Calories: 80
- Protein: 6g
- Fat: 4g
- Carbohydrates: 6g
- Fiber: 1g

## 31. Grilled Eggplant and Tomato Stacks with Basil Pesto

**Prep Time:** 15 minutes | **Cook Time:** 10 minutes | **Servings:** 4

### Ingredients:

- 2 medium eggplants, sliced into 1/2-inch rounds
- 2 large tomatoes, sliced
- For the Basil Pesto:
    - 1 cup fresh basil leaves
    - 1/4 cup pine nuts
    - 1/4 cup grated Parmesan cheese
    - 2 garlic cloves
    - 1/2 cup olive oil
    - Salt and pepper, to taste

### Directions:

1. Preheat grill to medium-high heat.
2. Grill eggplant slices for 3-4 minutes per side, until tender and grill marks appear.
3. For the pesto, blend basil leaves, pine nuts, Parmesan cheese, garlic, and olive oil in a food processor until smooth. Season with salt and pepper.

4. To assemble, layer an eggplant slice, a spoonful of basil pesto, and a tomato slice. Repeat the layering process until all ingredients are used.
5. Serve immediately, with extra basil pesto on the side.

**Nutritional Information:** (approximation)

- Calories: 280
- Protein: 5g
- Fat: 24g
- Carbohydrates: 12g
- Fiber: 6g

## 32. Moroccan Lentil and Vegetable Stew

**Prep Time:** 10 minutes | **Cook Time:** 35 minutes | **Servings:** 4

**Ingredients:**

- 1 tablespoon olive oil
- 1 onion, diced
- 2 carrots, diced
- 2 garlic cloves, minced
- 1 sweet potato, peeled and cubed
- 1 cup lentils, rinsed
- 4 cups vegetable broth

- 1 teaspoon ground cumin
- 1 teaspoon ground cinnamon
- 1/2 teaspoon ground turmeric
- 1/4 cup raisins
- Salt and pepper, to taste

**Directions:**

1. Heat olive oil in a large pot over medium heat. Add onion, carrots, and garlic. Sauté until softened, about 5 minutes.
2. Add sweet potato, lentils, vegetable broth, cumin, cinnamon, turmeric, raisins, salt, and pepper to the pot. Bring to a boil.
3. Reduce heat to low, cover, and simmer for 25-30 minutes, or until lentils and sweet potatoes are tender.
4. Adjust seasoning to taste. Serve hot, garnished with fresh cilantro if desired.

**Nutritional Information:** (approximation)

- Calories: 250
- Protein: 10g
- Fat: 4g
- Carbohydrates: 45g
- Fiber: 10g

## 33. Baked Cod with Lemon and Dill

**Prep Time:** 5 minutes | **Cook Time:** 15 minutes | **Servings:** 4

**Ingredients:**

- 4 cod fillets (6 ounces each)
- 2 tablespoons olive oil
- Juice of 1 lemon
- 1 tablespoon fresh dill, chopped
- Salt and pepper, to taste
- Lemon slices, for garnish

**Directions:**

1. Preheat oven to 400°F (200°C). Line a baking sheet with parchment paper.
2. Place cod fillets on the prepared baking sheet. Drizzle with olive oil and lemon juice. Season with salt, pepper, and dill.
3. Bake for 12-15 minutes, or until fish flakes easily with a fork.
4. Serve immediately, garnished with lemon slices and additional dill if desired.

**Nutritional Information:** (approximation)

- Calories: 180
- Protein: 23g
- Fat: 9g

- Carbohydrates: 1g
- Fiber: 0g

## 34. Kale Caesar Salad with Grilled Chicken

**Prep Time:** 20 minutes | **Cook Time:** 10 minutes | **Servings:** 4

**Ingredients:**

- 2 boneless, skinless chicken breasts
- Salt and pepper, to taste
- 1 tablespoon olive oil
- 4 cups kale, stems removed and leaves chopped
- For the Caesar Dressing:
    - 1/4 cup Greek yogurt
    - 1 tablespoon lemon juice
    - 1 teaspoon Dijon mustard
    - 1 garlic clove, minced
    - 2 tablespoons grated Parmesan cheese
    - 2 anchovy fillets, minced (optional)
    - Salt and pepper, to taste

**Directions:**

1. Season chicken breasts with salt and pepper. Heat olive oil in a grill pan over medium-high heat. Grill chicken for 5 minutes on each side, or until fully cooked. Let it rest for a few minutes before slicing.
2. In a large bowl, combine chopped kale and Caesar dressing ingredients. Toss until the kale is evenly coated with the dressing.
3. Add sliced grilled chicken on top of the kale.
4. Serve immediately, optionally garnished with additional Parmesan cheese and croutons.

**Nutritional Information:** (approximation)

- Calories: 250
- Protein: 28g
- Fat: 12g
- Carbohydrates: 8g
- Fiber: 2g

### 35. Butternut Squash and Spinach Lasagna

**Prep Time:** 30 minutes | **Cook Time:** 45 minutes | **Servings:** 6

**Ingredients:**

- 1 butternut squash, peeled, seeded, and sliced
- 2 cups spinach, washed

- 1 cup ricotta cheese
- 1/2 cup grated Parmesan cheese
- 1 egg
- Salt and pepper, to taste
- 9 gluten-free lasagna noodles, cooked
- 2 cups marinara sauce

**Directions:**

1. Preheat oven to 375°F (190°C).
2. In a bowl, mix ricotta cheese, Parmesan cheese, egg, salt, and pepper.
3. Spread a thin layer of marinara sauce on the bottom of a baking dish.
4. Layer the dish with lasagna noodles, followed by the ricotta mixture, slices of butternut squash, spinach, and more marinara sauce. Repeat the layers until all ingredients are used, finishing with a layer of marinara sauce.
5. Cover with aluminum foil and bake for 30 minutes. Remove foil and bake for an additional 15 minutes, or until the top is golden and bubbly.
6. Let it cool for 10 minutes before serving.

**Nutritional Information:** (approximation)

- Calories: 350
- Protein: 15g

- Fat: 12g
- Carbohydrates: 45g
- Fiber: 5g

## 36. Asian-Inspired Beef and Broccoli Stir-Fry

**Prep Time:** 15 minutes | **Cook Time:** 10 minutes | **Servings:** 4

**Ingredients:**

- 1 pound (450g) beef sirloin, thinly sliced
- 2 tablespoons soy sauce
- 1 tablespoon sesame oil
- 2 cups broccoli florets
- 1 garlic clove, minced
- 1 inch ginger, minced
- 1 tablespoon olive oil
- 2 tablespoons oyster sauce
- 1 teaspoon cornstarch dissolved in 2 tablespoons water

**Directions:**

1. In a bowl, marinate the beef slices in soy sauce and sesame oil for at least 15 minutes.

2. Heat olive oil in a large skillet or wok over high heat. Add garlic and ginger; stir-fry for 30 seconds.

3. Add the marinated beef and stir-fry for 2-3 minutes, or until it starts to brown.

4. Add broccoli florets and continue to stir-fry for another 3-4 minutes, or until the broccoli is tender but still crisp.

5. Stir in oyster sauce and the cornstarch mixture. Cook until the sauce thickens, about 1-2 minutes.

6. Serve immediately, over a bed of cooked rice or noodles if desired.

**Nutritional Information:** (approximation)

- Calories: 300
- Protein: 26g
- Fat: 18g
- Carbohydrates: 8g
- Fiber: 2g"

# Snacks

### 37. Avocado and Chickpea Hummus Dip

"**Prep Time:** 10 minutes | **Cook Time:** 0 minutes | **Servings:** 4

**Ingredients:**

- 1 ripe avocado
- 1 can (15 oz) chickpeas, drained and rinsed
- Juice of 1 lemon
- 2 cloves garlic, minced
- Salt and pepper, to taste
- 2 tablespoons extra virgin olive oil
- Water, as needed

**Directions:**

1. In a food processor, blend avocado, chickpeas, lemon juice, garlic, salt, and pepper until smooth.
2. While processing, gradually add olive oil and water as needed to achieve a creamy consistency.
3. Adjust seasoning to taste. Serve with raw vegetables or whole-grain crackers.

**Nutritional Information:** (approximation)

- Calories: 220
- Protein: 7g
- Fat: 14g
- Carbohydrates: 20g
- Fiber: 8g

## 38. Golden Turmeric and Almond Milk Smoothie

**Prep Time:** 5 minutes | **Cook Time:** 0 minutes | **Servings:** 2

**Ingredients:**

- 1 cup unsweetened almond milk
- 1 banana, frozen
- 1/2 teaspoon ground turmeric
- 1/4 teaspoon ground cinnamon
- 1 tablespoon honey (optional)

**Directions:**

1. Combine almond milk, banana, turmeric, cinnamon, and honey (if using) in a blender.
2. Blend until smooth and creamy.
3. Serve immediately, garnished with a sprinkle of cinnamon.

**Nutritional Information:** (approximation)

- Calories: 150
- Protein: 2g
- Fat: 3g
- Carbohydrates: 30g
- Fiber: 4g

## 39. Kale Chips with Sea Salt

**Prep Time:** 10 minutes | **Cook Time:** 15 minutes | **Servings:** 4

**Ingredients:**

- 1 bunch kale, stems removed and leaves torn into bite-sized pieces
- 1 tablespoon olive oil
- Sea salt, to taste

**Directions:**

1. Preheat oven to 300°F (150°C). Line a baking sheet with parchment paper.
2. Toss kale leaves with olive oil and spread in a single layer on the baking sheet.
3. Sprinkle with sea salt.
4. Bake for 15 minutes, or until crisp, turning halfway through.
5. Let cool before serving.

**Nutritional Information:** (approximation)

- Calories: 80
- Protein: 2g
- Fat: 5g
- Carbohydrates: 7g
- Fiber: 2g

## 40. Chia Seed Pudding with Mixed Berries

**Prep Time:** 8 hours (overnight) | **Cook Time:** 0 minutes | **Servings:** 2

**Ingredients:**

- 1/4 cup chia seeds
- 1 cup unsweetened almond milk
- 1 tablespoon maple syrup (optional)
- 1/2 cup mixed berries

**Directions:**

1. In a bowl, mix chia seeds, almond milk, and maple syrup (if using).
2. Cover and refrigerate overnight.
3. Before serving, stir the pudding and top with mixed berries.

**Nutritional Information:** (approximation)

- Calories: 200
- Protein: 5g
- Fat: 10g
- Carbohydrates: 24g
- Fiber: 10g

Given the detailed nature of these recipes, I'll continue with the remaining snack recipes in the next response to ensure each one is comprehensive and beginner-friendly. Let's proceed with the next set.

Continuing with the detailed snack recipes:

### 41. Spiced Roasted Nuts

**Prep Time:** 5 minutes | **Cook Time:** 10 minutes | **Servings:** 4

**Ingredients:**

- 2 cups mixed nuts (almonds, walnuts, cashews)
- 1 tablespoon olive oil
- 1 teaspoon ground turmeric
- 1/2 teaspoon ground cinnamon
- 1/4 teaspoon cayenne pepper (optional)
- Salt, to taste

**Directions:**

1. Preheat the oven to 350°F (175°C). Line a baking sheet with parchment paper.
2. In a bowl, toss the nuts with olive oil, turmeric, cinnamon, cayenne pepper (if using), and salt until well coated.
3. Spread the nuts in a single layer on the prepared baking sheet.
4. Bake for 10 minutes, or until golden and fragrant. Stir halfway through to ensure even roasting.

5. Cool before serving. Store in an airtight container.

**Nutritional Information:** (approximation)

- Calories: 300
- Protein: 8g
- Fat: 26g
- Carbohydrates: 12g
- Fiber: 4g

## 42. Carrot and Cucumber Sticks with Almond Butter Dip

**Prep Time:** 10 minutes | **Cook Time:** 0 minutes | **Servings:** 4

**Ingredients:**

- 2 large carrots, peeled and cut into sticks
- 1 large cucumber, cut into sticks
- 1/2 cup almond butter
- 2 tablespoons lemon juice
- 1 tablespoon honey (optional)
- Pinch of salt

**Directions:**

1. In a small bowl, mix almond butter, lemon juice, honey (if using), and a pinch of salt until

smooth. Adjust consistency with a little water if needed.

2. Serve carrot and cucumber sticks alongside the almond butter dip.

**Nutritional Information:** (approximation)

- Calories: 220
- Protein: 6g
- Fat: 16g
- Carbohydrates: 16g
- Fiber: 4g

## 43. Baked Sweet Potato Wedges

**Prep Time:** 10 minutes | **Cook Time:** 25 minutes | **Servings:** 4

**Ingredients:**

- 2 large sweet potatoes, cut into wedges
- 2 tablespoons olive oil
- 1 teaspoon smoked paprika
- Salt and pepper, to taste

**Directions:**

1. Preheat the oven to 400°F (200°C). Line a baking sheet with parchment paper.

2. Toss sweet potato wedges with olive oil, smoked paprika, salt, and pepper.
3. Arrange the wedges in a single layer on the baking sheet.
4. Bake for 25 minutes, or until tender and crispy. Turn once halfway through cooking.
5. Serve warm.

**Nutritional Information:** (approximation)

- Calories: 180
- Protein: 2g
- Fat: 7g
- Carbohydrates: 27g
- Fiber: 4g

## 44. Zucchini and Carrot Fritters

**Prep Time:** 20 minutes | **Cook Time:** 10 minutes | **Servings:** 4

**Ingredients:**

- 1 zucchini, grated
- 2 carrots, grated
- 2 eggs
- 1/4 cup almond flour
- 1/2 teaspoon garlic powder

- Salt and pepper, to taste
- Olive oil for frying

**Directions:**

1. Squeeze the grated zucchini and carrots to remove excess moisture.
2. In a bowl, mix the zucchini, carrots, eggs, almond flour, garlic powder, salt, and pepper.
3. Heat olive oil in a skillet over medium heat. Scoop spoonfuls of the mixture into the skillet, flattening to form fritters.
4. Fry for 3-4 minutes on each side, until golden and crispy.
5. Drain on paper towels and serve warm.

**Nutritional Information:** (approximation)

- Calories: 150
- Protein: 6g
- Fat: 11g
- Carbohydrates: 8g
- Fiber: 3g

## 45. Apple Slices with Cinnamon and Nutmeg

**Prep Time:** 5 minutes | **Cook Time:** 0 minutes | **Servings:** 4

**Ingredients:**

- 2 large apples, cored and sliced
- 1/2 teaspoon ground cinnamon
- 1/4 teaspoon ground nutmeg

**Directions:**

1. Arrange apple slices on a serving plate.
2. Sprinkle evenly with ground cinnamon and nutmeg.
3. Serve immediately, or refrigerate until ready to eat. Enjoy as a fresh, crunchy snack.

**Nutritional Information:** (approximation)

- Calories: 50
- Protein: 0g
- Fat: 0g
- Carbohydrates: 13g
- Fiber: 2g

## 46. Beetroot and Ginger Juice

**Prep Time:** 10 minutes | **Cook Time:** 0 minutes | **Servings:** 2

**Ingredients:**

- 2 medium beetroots, peeled and chopped
- 1 inch ginger, peeled
- 1 apple, cored and chopped

- 1/2 lemon, juiced

**Directions:**

1. Place beetroot, ginger, and apple in a juicer. Process until smooth.
2. Stir in lemon juice.
3. Serve immediately, over ice if desired, for a refreshing and invigorating drink.

**Nutritional Information:** (approximation)

- Calories: 100
- Protein: 2g
- Fat: 0g
- Carbohydrates: 25g
- Fiber: 6g

## 47. Pumpkin Seed and Cranberry Energy Bars

**Prep Time:** 15 minutes | **Cook Time:** 20 minutes | **Servings:** 8

**Ingredients:**

- 1 cup oats
- 1/2 cup pumpkin seeds
- 1/2 cup dried cranberries
- 1/4 cup honey or maple syrup

- 1/4 cup almond butter
- 1 teaspoon vanilla extract
- Pinch of salt

**Directions:**

1. Preheat the oven to 350°F (175°C). Line an 8x8 inch baking dish with parchment paper.
2. In a large bowl, mix oats, pumpkin seeds, and dried cranberries.
3. In a small saucepan, warm honey (or maple syrup) and almond butter over low heat until smoothly combined. Stir in vanilla extract and salt.
4. Pour the liquid mixture over the dry ingredients and stir until well combined.
5. Press the mixture firmly into the prepared baking dish.
6. Bake for 20 minutes, or until the edges are golden brown.
7. Cool completely before cutting into bars.

**Nutritional Information:** (approximation)

- Calories: 200
- Protein: 5g
- Fat: 10g
- Carbohydrates: 25g
- Fiber: 3g

## 48. Cauliflower Buffalo Bites

**Prep Time:** 15 minutes | **Cook Time:** 25 minutes | **Servings:** 4

**Ingredients:**

- 1 head cauliflower, cut into bite-sized florets
- 1/2 cup all-purpose flour (or almond flour for gluten-free option)
- 1/2 cup water
- 1 teaspoon garlic powder
- Salt and pepper, to taste
- 1/2 cup buffalo sauce
- 1 tablespoon olive oil

**Directions:**

1. Preheat the oven to 450°F (230°C). Line a baking sheet with parchment paper.
2. In a large bowl, whisk together flour, water, garlic powder, salt, and pepper. Add cauliflower florets and toss until well coated.
3. Spread cauliflower in a single layer on the baking sheet. Bake for 20 minutes, flipping halfway through.
4. In a small bowl, mix buffalo sauce with olive oil. Toss baked cauliflower in the sauce.

5. Return cauliflower to the oven and bake for an additional 5 minutes.
6. Serve hot with dairy-free ranch dressing for dipping.

**Nutritional Information:** (approximation)
- Calories: 150
- Protein: 4g
- Fat: 5g
- Carbohydrates: 22g
- Fiber: 3g"

# Desserts

### 49. Ginger-Spiced Apple Crisp

"**Prep Time:** 15 minutes | **Cook Time:** 30 minutes | **Servings:** 6

**Ingredients:**
- 4 large apples, peeled, cored, and sliced
- 1 teaspoon ground cinnamon
- 1/2 teaspoon ground ginger
- 2 tablespoons maple syrup
- **For the topping:**
    - 1 cup almond flour
    - 1/2 cup rolled oats

- 1/4 cup coconut oil, melted
- 1/4 cup maple syrup
- 1/2 teaspoon vanilla extract
- Pinch of salt

**Directions:**

1. Preheat the oven to 350°F (175°C). In a large bowl, mix the apple slices with cinnamon, ginger, and maple syrup. Transfer to a baking dish.
2. In a separate bowl, combine almond flour, oats, coconut oil, maple syrup, vanilla, and salt for the topping. Mix until crumbly.
3. Sprinkle the topping over the apples in the baking dish.
4. Bake for 30 minutes or until the topping is golden and the apples are tender.
5. Serve warm, optionally with a dollop of dairy-free vanilla ice cream.

**Nutritional Information:** (approximation)

- Calories: 320
- Protein: 4g
- Fat: 18g
- Carbohydrates: 36g
- Fiber: 6g

## 50. Turmeric Coconut Milk Pudding

**Prep Time:** 5 minutes | **Cook Time:** 10 minutes | **Chill Time:** 2 hours | **Servings:** 4

### Ingredients:

- 1 can (13.5 oz) full-fat coconut milk
- 2 teaspoons ground turmeric
- 1/4 cup honey
- 1/4 cup water
- 2 teaspoons agar agar powder

### Directions:

1. In a saucepan, whisk together coconut milk, turmeric, honey, water, and agar agar.
2. Bring to a simmer over medium heat, stirring constantly, until the mixture thickens slightly, about 5-10 minutes.
3. Pour into serving dishes and chill in the refrigerator until set, about 2 hours.
4. Serve chilled, garnished with a sprinkle of cinnamon or sliced almonds if desired.

**Nutritional Information:** (approximation)

- Calories: 250
- Protein: 2g
- Fat: 22g
- Carbohydrates: 14g

- Fiber: 0g

## 51. Blueberry Lemon Chia Seed Parfait

**Prep Time:** 15 minutes (plus chilling time) | **Cook Time:** 0 minutes | **Servings:** 4

**Ingredients:**

- 1/4 cup chia seeds
- 1 cup unsweetened almond milk
- 2 tablespoons lemon juice
- Zest of 1 lemon
- 1 tablespoon maple syrup (adjust to taste)
- 1 cup fresh blueberries
- 1/4 cup crushed nuts (almonds or walnuts)

**Directions:**

1. In a bowl, combine chia seeds, almond milk, lemon juice, lemon zest, and maple syrup. Whisk until well combined.
2. Cover and refrigerate for at least 4 hours, or overnight, until the chia seeds have absorbed the liquid and the mixture has a pudding-like consistency.
3. To assemble the parfaits, layer the chia pudding with fresh blueberries and crushed nuts in serving glasses.

4. Serve chilled, garnished with extra lemon zest if desired.

**Nutritional Information:** (approximation)

- Calories: 180
- Protein: 4g
- Fat: 10g
- Carbohydrates: 20g
- Fiber: 7g

## 52. Dark Chocolate and Almond Butter Cups

**Prep Time:** 15 minutes | **Cook Time:** 0 minutes (plus freezing time) | **Servings:** 12 cups

**Ingredients:**

- 1 cup dark chocolate chips (at least 70% cocoa)
- 1/2 cup almond butter
- 2 tablespoons maple syrup
- Sea salt, for sprinkling

**Directions:**

1. Melt dark chocolate chips in a microwave-safe bowl or over a double boiler, stirring until smooth.

2. Pour a spoonful of melted chocolate into the bottom of silicone muffin cups or lined muffin tin, just enough to cover the base.
3. Freeze for 10 minutes until set.
4. Mix almond butter with maple syrup. Place a small spoonful of the almond butter mixture over the set chocolate base.
5. Cover the almond butter with another layer of melted chocolate, ensuring the almond butter is completely sealed.
6. Sprinkle a little sea salt on top of each cup.
7. Freeze for another 20 minutes or until firm. Remove from molds and store in an airtight container in the fridge.

**Nutritional Information:** (approximation)

- Calories: 150
- Protein: 3g
- Fat: 11g
- Carbohydrates: 12g
- Fiber: 2g

## 53. Avocado Chocolate Mousse

**Prep Time:** 10 minutes | **Cook Time:** 0 minutes | **Servings:** 4

**Ingredients:**

- 2 ripe avocados, pitted and scooped
- 1/4 cup cocoa powder
- 1/4 cup maple syrup (adjust to taste)
- 1 teaspoon vanilla extract
- Pinch of salt
- 1/4 cup almond milk (adjust for desired consistency)

**Directions:**

1. Combine avocados, cocoa powder, maple syrup, vanilla extract, salt, and almond milk in a blender or food processor. Blend until smooth and creamy.
2. Adjust sweetness with more maple syrup if needed. If the mousse is too thick, add a little more almond milk to reach the desired consistency.
3. Chill in the refrigerator for at least 1 hour before serving.
4. Serve garnished with fresh berries or a sprinkle of cocoa powder.

**Nutritional Information:** (approximation)

- Calories: 250
- Protein: 4g
- Fat: 18g
- Carbohydrates: 24g

- Fiber: 7g

### 54. Sweet Potato Brownies

**Prep Time:** 15 minutes | **Cook Time:** 25 minutes | **Servings:** 8

**Ingredients:**

- 1 cup sweet potato puree
- 1/2 cup almond flour
- 1/2 cup cocoa powder
- 1/2 cup maple syrup
- 1/4 cup coconut oil, melted
- 1 teaspoon vanilla extract
- 1/2 teaspoon baking powder
- Pinch of salt

**Directions:**

1. Preheat the oven to 350°F (175°C). Line an 8x8 inch baking dish with parchment paper.
2. In a large bowl, combine sweet potato puree, almond flour, cocoa powder, maple syrup, coconut oil, vanilla extract, baking powder, and salt. Mix until well combined.
3. Pour the batter into the prepared baking dish, smoothing the top with a spatula.

4. Bake for 25 minutes, or until a toothpick inserted into the center comes out clean.

5. Let cool before cutting into squares and serving.

**Nutritional Information:** (approximation)

- Calories: 200
- Protein: 3g
- Fat: 11g
- Carbohydrates: 25g
- Fiber: 4g

## 55. Carrot Cake Energy Balls

**Prep Time:** 20 minutes | **Cook Time:** 0 minutes | **Servings:** 12 balls

**Ingredients:**

- 1 cup shredded carrots
- 1 cup dates, pitted
- 1/2 cup walnuts
- 1/2 cup unsweetened shredded coconut, plus extra for rolling
- 1 teaspoon cinnamon
- 1/4 teaspoon nutmeg
- Pinch of salt

**Directions:**

1. In a food processor, combine shredded carrots, dates, walnuts, shredded coconut, cinnamon, nutmeg, and salt. Process until the mixture sticks together.
2. Roll the mixture into balls, about 1 inch in diameter.
3. Roll the balls in additional shredded coconut to coat.
4. Chill in the refrigerator for at least 1 hour before serving. Store in an airtight container in the fridge.

**Nutritional Information:** (approximation)

- Calories: 120
- Protein: 2g
- Fat: 7g
- Carbohydrates: 14g
- Fiber: 3g

## 56. Baked Pears with Honey and Walnuts

**Prep Time:** 10 minutes | **Cook Time:** 25 minutes | **Servings:** 4

**Ingredients:**

- 2 large pears, halved and cored

- 2 tablespoons honey
- 1/4 cup walnuts, chopped
- 1/2 teaspoon cinnamon

**Directions:**

1. Preheat the oven to 350°F (175°C). Place pear halves, cut-side up, in a baking dish.
2. Drizzle honey over pears, then sprinkle with chopped walnuts and cinnamon.
3. Bake for 25 minutes, or until pears are tender and walnuts are toasted.
4. Serve warm, possibly with a dollop of Greek yogurt.

**Nutritional Information:** (approximation)

- Calories: 150
- Protein: 2g
- Fat: 5g
- Carbohydrates: 27g
- Fiber: 4g

## 57. Raspberry and Almond Flour Scones

**Prep Time:** 15 minutes | **Cook Time:** 20 minutes | **Servings:** 8 scones

**Ingredients:**

- 2 cups almond flour
- 1/3 cup fresh raspberries
- 1/4 cup honey or maple syrup
- 1 egg
- 1 teaspoon vanilla extract
- 1/2 teaspoon baking soda
- Pinch of salt

**Directions:**

1. Preheat the oven to 350°F (175°C) and line a baking sheet with parchment paper.
2. In a large bowl, mix almond flour, baking soda, and salt. Add honey, egg, and vanilla extract, mixing until well combined.
3. Gently fold in raspberries.
4. Form the dough into a circle on the prepared baking sheet, then cut into 8 wedges.
5. Bake for 20 minutes, or until golden brown.
6. Let cool before serving.

**Nutritional Information:** (approximation)

- Calories: 220
- Protein: 6g
- Fat: 16g
- Carbohydrates: 16g
- Fiber: 4g

## 58. Mango Coconut Ice Cream

**Prep Time:** 10 minutes (plus freezing time) | **Cook Time:** 0 minutes | **Servings:** 4

**Ingredients:**

- 2 cups ripe mango, cubed
- 1 can (13.5 oz) full-fat coconut milk
- 1/4 cup honey or maple syrup
- 1 teaspoon lime zest

**Directions:**

1. Blend mango, coconut milk, honey, and lime zest in a blender until smooth.
2. Pour mixture into an ice cream maker and churn according to the manufacturer's instructions.
3. Transfer to a freezer-safe container and freeze until firm, about 4 hours.
4. Let sit at room temperature for a few minutes before scooping and serving.

**Nutritional Information:** (approximation)

- Calories: 300
- Protein: 3g
- Fat: 20g
- Carbohydrates: 30g

- Fiber: 2g

## 59. Pumpkin Spice Chia Pudding

**Prep Time:** 10 minutes (plus chilling time) | **Cook Time:** 0 minutes | **Servings:** 4

**Ingredients:**

- 1/4 cup chia seeds
- 1 cup unsweetened almond milk
- 1/2 cup pumpkin puree
- 2 tablespoons maple syrup (adjust to taste)
- 1 teaspoon pumpkin pie spice
- 1/4 cup pecans, chopped

**Directions:**

1. In a mixing bowl, whisk together the chia seeds, almond milk, pumpkin puree, maple syrup, and pumpkin pie spice until well combined.
2. Divide the mixture evenly into serving glasses or bowls. Cover and refrigerate for at least 4 hours, or overnight, until the pudding has thickened and the chia seeds have absorbed the liquid.
3. Before serving, stir the pudding to check consistency. If it's too thick, you can thin it with a little more almond milk.

4. Top each serving with chopped pecans for added crunch.

5. Serve chilled as a delicious fall-inspired dessert or breakfast.

**Nutritional Information:** (approximation)

- Calories: 180
- Protein: 4g
- Fat: 10g
- Carbohydrates: 20g
- Fiber: 6g

### 60. Zucchini Chocolate Chip Cookies

**Prep Time:** 15 minutes | **Cook Time:** 12 minutes | **Servings:** 12 cookies

**Ingredients:**

- 1 cup almond flour
- 1/2 cup grated zucchini, squeezed of excess moisture
- 1/4 cup dark chocolate chips
- 1/4 cup maple syrup
- 1 egg
- 1 teaspoon vanilla extract
- 1/2 teaspoon baking soda

- Pinch of salt

**Directions:**

1. Preheat the oven to 350°F (175°C). Line a baking sheet with parchment paper.
2. In a large bowl, combine almond flour, baking soda, and salt.
3. In another bowl, mix the grated zucchini, maple syrup, egg, and vanilla extract until well combined.
4. Add the wet ingredients to the dry ingredients, mixing until just combined. Fold in the chocolate chips.
5. Drop tablespoonfuls of the dough onto the prepared baking sheet, spacing them about 2 inches apart.
6. Bake for 12 minutes, or until the edges are golden brown and the centers have set.
7. Let the cookies cool on the baking sheet for 5 minutes before transferring them to a wire rack to cool completely.
8. Enjoy a deliciously moist and flavorful treat that sneaks in some veggies!

**Nutritional Information:** (approximation)

- Calories: 120
- Protein: 3g
- Fat: 8g

- Carbohydrates: 10g
- Fiber: 2g"

*Chapter 4*

# 7-Day Meal Plan

"**Day 1:**
- **Breakfast:** Golden Turmeric and Almond Milk Smoothie
- **Lunch:** Mediterranean Quinoa Salad
- **Snack:** Avocado and Chickpea Hummus Dip with Vegetable Sticks
- **Dinner:** Ginger-Spiced Apple Crisp
- **Dessert:** Pumpkin Spice Chia Pudding

**Day 2:**
- **Breakfast:** Chia Seed Pudding with Mixed Berries
- **Lunch:** Turmeric Chicken Wraps
- **Snack:** Carrot and Cucumber Sticks with Almond Butter Dip
- **Dinner:** Zucchini and Carrot Fritters with a side of Baked Sweet Potato Wedges
- **Dessert:** Avocado Chocolate Mousse

**Day 3:**
- **Breakfast:** Blueberry Lemon Chia Seed Parfait

- **Lunch:** Spicy Sweet Potato and Black Bean Chili
- **Snack:** Spiced Roasted Nuts
- **Dinner:** Turmeric Roasted Chicken and Vegetables
- **Dessert:** Sweet Potato Brownies

**Day 4:**
- **Breakfast:** Apple Slices with Cinnamon and Nutmeg
- **Lunch:** Grilled Vegetable and Hummus Flatbread
- **Snack:** Kale Chips with Sea Salt
- **Dinner:** Lemon Garlic Shrimp with Zucchini Noodles
- **Dessert:** Raspberry and Almond Flour Scones

**Day 5:**
- **Breakfast:** Pumpkin Seed and Cranberry Energy Bars
- **Lunch:** Moroccan Lentil and Vegetable Stew
- **Snack:** Baked Pears with Honey and Walnuts
- **Dinner:** Baked Cod with Lemon and Dill
- **Dessert:** Dark Chocolate and Almond Butter Cups

**Day 6:**

- **Breakfast:** Mango Coconut Ice Cream (as a smoothie bowl topped with granola)
- **Lunch:** Stuffed Bell Peppers with Quinoa and Ground Turkey
- **Snack:** Roasted Chickpeas
- **Dinner:** Asian-Inspired Beef and Broccoli Stir-Fry
- **Dessert:** Carrot Cake Energy Balls

**Day 7:**

- **Breakfast:** Beetroot and Ginger Juice with a side of Flaxseed Crackers
- **Lunch:** Kale Caesar Salad with Grilled Chicken
- **Snack:** Zucchini Chocolate Chip Cookies
- **Dinner:** Miso Soup with Tofu and Seaweed followed by Grilled Eggplant and Tomato Stacks with Basil Pesto
- **Dessert:** Ginger Pear Compote (served over Greek yogurt or dairy-free alternative)"

*Chapter 5*

# Lifestyle Changes to Complement Your Diet

"Adopting an anti-inflammatory diet is a pivotal step towards enhancing your health, reducing pain, and revitalizing your energy levels. However, to fully harness the benefits of this dietary approach, it's crucial to complement it with positive lifestyle changes. This chapter focuses on holistic wellness by integrating suitable exercise routines, effective stress management techniques, and strategies to improve sleep quality.

## Exercise routines suitable for all levels

Exercise plays a vital role in reducing inflammation and improving overall well-being. It can boost your mood, enhance your cardiovascular health, and strengthen your muscles and joints. Here are some exercise routines suitable for all fitness levels:

- **Walking:** A simple yet effective low-impact exercise that can be easily incorporated into your daily routine. Aim for at least 30 minutes of brisk walking most days of the week.

- **Yoga:** Offers a combination of physical postures, breathing exercises, and meditation to reduce stress, improve flexibility, and lower inflammation. Start with gentle yoga classes or online sessions designed for beginners.
- **Swimming:** An excellent full-body workout that minimizes stress on the joints, making it ideal for individuals with joint pain or arthritis.
- **Strength Training:** Building muscle can help regulate blood sugar levels, reduce fat, and combat inflammation. Use light weights or resistance bands, focusing on major muscle groups. Begin with one set of exercises, gradually increasing the weight and number of sets as you become stronger.

## Stress management techniques

Stress can exacerbate inflammation and negatively impact your health. Incorporating stress reduction techniques into your daily life can significantly enhance your dietary efforts:

- **Mindfulness Meditation:** Dedicate a few minutes each day to mindfulness, focusing on your breath and the present moment to reduce stress and anxiety.

- **Deep Breathing Exercises:** Practice deep breathing techniques, such as diaphragmatic breathing, to calm the nervous system and reduce stress levels.
- **Time in Nature:** Spending time outdoors, especially in green spaces, can lower stress hormones and promote a sense of well-being.
- **Hobbies:** Engage in activities you enjoy, whether it's reading, gardening, painting, or listening to music, to distract from stressors and relax your mind.

## Importance of sleep and how to improve sleep quality

Sleep is essential for healing, immune function, and reducing inflammation. Poor sleep quality can undermine the benefits of a healthy diet. Here are strategies to improve your sleep:

- **Consistent Sleep Schedule:** Try to go to bed and wake up at the same time every day, even on weekends, to regulate your body's internal clock.
- **Create a Restful Environment:** Ensure your bedroom is quiet, dark, and cool. Consider using blackout curtains, earplugs, or white noise machines if necessary.

- **Limit Screen Time:** Reduce exposure to screens at least an hour before bedtime, as the blue light emitted can disrupt your body's natural sleep-wake cycle.
- **Relaxation Techniques:** Incorporate relaxation practices before bed, such as reading, taking a warm bath, or gentle stretching, to prepare your body for sleep.

Combining an anti-inflammatory diet with these lifestyle changes can significantly enhance your health and well-being. Remember, small, consistent adjustments can lead to profound long-term benefits. Embrace these practices to complement your dietary efforts and achieve optimal health."

# **Conclusion**

Reaching the end of this cookbook marks the beginning of a transformative journey towards improved health and well-being. This cookbook was crafted not merely as a compilation of recipes but as a holistic guide aimed at reducing inflammation through dietary choices and lifestyle modifications.

By incorporating the principles of an anti-inflammatory diet, engaging in the beginner-friendly recipes provided, and adhering to the suggested lifestyle changes, you are taking a comprehensive approach to health. This approach addresses inflammation at its core, offering a pathway to healing and vitality. From nourishing breakfasts to satisfying dinners, each recipe is designed not only to delight the palate but also to promote your body's natural healing processes.

The path to wellness extends beyond the kitchen. Regular physical activity, effective stress management, and prioritizing sleep are essential components of a balanced lifestyle. These elements work in concert with dietary choices to combat inflammation and enhance overall well-being. They are key to improving your energy levels, mental clarity, and quality of life.

Transitioning to an anti-inflammatory lifestyle is a personal and gradual process that requires dedication and patience. Embrace small, consistent steps toward making healthier choices, and remember that every change contributes to a larger impact on your health. It's important to listen to your body, practice self-compassion, and seek support when needed.

We hope this cookbook becomes a cherished resource on your journey toward health and vitality. Let the recipes and guidance within these pages inspire you to adopt a lifestyle that nourishes and rejuvenates. Cheers to a healthier, more vibrant you!

Thank you for allowing this book to be part of your journey toward a healthier life.

Made in the USA
Las Vegas, NV
25 July 2024